Dental Practice F

Policies & Procedures

By Drs. Lovell & Schwindt

C 2013

Dental Practice

Resource

Group

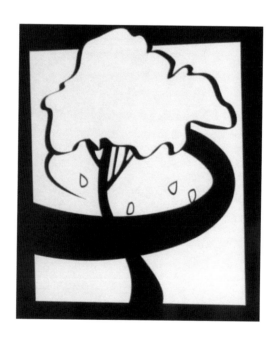

Dental Office Employee Manual

Policies & Procedures

DentalPracticeResourceGroup.com

Dental Practice Resource Group

About Us

Dental Practice Resource Group was formed with the sole mission of helping busy dental practices solve their practice related issues. Our team members have been practicing and collaborating on various projects over the last two decades and have come under the same umbrella a few years ago. We are very excited to have merged with Singularis Media Group and now have expanded our services. We have been using Singularis Media Group's web services for SEO, link building and video marketing for the last two years so the partnership was the next logical progression.

As busy clinicians it is very difficult to find the time to develop policies and procedures from scratch. Why reinvent the wheel? Dentistry at its core is the same wherever it is practiced; however, the nuances of practice management and marketing are what set apart the most successful dentists.

Our mission was to create a series of resources on a wide variety of topics specific to the dental office. Over the last year, we have been refining these resources and making them available to our fellow colleagues in the dental industry. We strive to make these resources valuable yet clean and simple. We have been told that their format allows for easy modification and customization based on the dental practice that utilizes them. With that in mind, we are making all of our resources available in a variety of formats (PDF, eBook, MS Word, RTF). Several of these formats lend for modification and can be tailored to any dental practice needs.

Our team is fortunate to have the input of a physician who shares a unique perspective on the issues at the crossroads of both dentistry and medicine. For that reason, we believe that our resources have a distinct advantage over what is otherwise available. Our business model is centered around a dental office and all of these resources and web-based strategies have been implemented in our own practice. Our team consists of dedicated health professionals who happen to be passionate about dental marketing and education.

Being a dentist and transforming lives (and smiles) has never been more rewarding. We know you will find value in this resource. Visit our website and see what else we have to offer.

DentalPracticeResourceGroup.com

Table Of Contents:

Other Publications by Dental Practice Resource Group

Managing Medical Emergencies In The Dental Office

The Comprehensive Dental Practice Guide

Available on Amazon, Barnes & Nobel, Kobo, Smashwords and more.

For other format options, please visit our website:

DentalPracticeResourceGroup.com

The information contained within is what we use in our practice and office management strategy. We thought: "Why reinvent the wheel?" By sharing the tools we have developed over the last

15 years we hope to simplify the approach to common issues for the dental office. We make our disclaimer here that no guarantee of any sort exists and the reader/user takes it upon themselves to adapt, modify and research how to best implement a strategy that makes practical sense for their unique situation. We are not giving legal, accounting, dental or medical advice but only put forth these guides to share knowledge and hope that in doing so it will free up time for the dentist or office manager to focus on what matters the most – the patients!

Dental Practice Resource Group

Employee Manual

Policy Overview

Mission Statement

Employee Manual

This is the new employee handbook we have developed for use and modification. We have taken this template and expanded it for each of the practice locations. If you would like this in a MS Word format for modification please let us know or locate it on the website (DentalPracticeResourceGroup.com).

The terms used to identify a practice, dentist and employee were purposely left generic to allow this manual to stand alone as is without significant modification or to serve as a working template to create a unique manual customized for any practice needs.

Why reinvent the wheel? If your office does not have such a manual or you are just starting your very first practice or perhaps opening a new office, Dental Practice Resource Group has the resources and tools to make your life easier.

Please review the details contained within this document, as certain aspects will require change: office hours, time off, paid CE, etc.

Look for our other manuals on common office issues such as: OSHA, Radiation

Safety, Exposure to blood and body fluids and more.

Wishing you the best,

The Team at Dental Practice Resource Group

Welcome

Welcome to our practice! Our goal is to develop a welcoming, positive, and friendly working atmosphere. We will strive daily to create a comfortable and professionally challenging environment that you will feel at home in. The welfare of our patients and practice is dependent on a happy, cooperative and effective staff.

As an employee, this is your manual of office policies and procedures. This employee manual is not an expressed or implied contract of employment. We reserve the right to change, modify, or delete any provision of this manual at our sole discretion with or without notice. Either this dental office or employee may terminate the employment relationship at any time with or without notice or cause. This manual will be given to and reviewed with each and every employee. The employee will be expected to acknowledge that this was completed with a signed statement. This manual will be reviewed on an annual basis at minimum. Please bring any questions or concerns to our attention anytime an issue or concern arises.

Our Mission:

To improve the lives of our patients by providing comprehensive dental care and education at a fair fee with a priority given to patient comfort, efficiency of service and positive dental experiences. To welcome patients into an environment that is personal, relaxing and calm, to insure their comfort within all areas of the practice.

Within this Mission Statement:

1. Provide a safe, enjoyable, positive atmosphere for all employees. Encourage employees to be highly motivated and willing to grow in

their professions. To provide a fair wage and benefit package for employees which is outlined in an at-will contract.

2. Provide all of our patient's treatment in a polite, kind, and empathetic manner. To promote regular preventative care, both at home and at our office encouraging optimum oral health.

3. To provide dental care in a state-of-the–art facility, striving to remain current with the latest technology, equipment, materials, and education. To encourage staff to promote our dedication to this area, take ample continuing education, and to take care of and maintain our resources.

OPEN DOOR POLICY:

This office has an Open Door Policy and encourages employees to bring their concerns to the management for resolution. We know that problems can occur at any organization including interpretation of policies or other disagreements. Feel free to communicate your comments to us either verbally or in writing. We want you to enjoy your workplace! The dental office manager is generally the first point of contact, but feel free to discuss your concerns with any of the staff dentists.

NEW HIRE CHECKLIST:

Within the first week of employment of any new employee a "New Hire Checklist" will be completed with the new employee. This checklist is a tool used to orient the new employee to all office policies and procedures, collect necessary paperwork and documentation, and to go over wage, PTO, unpaid leave, benefits, office hours, dress and appearance expectations, attendance policy, work schedule, job description, etc. This is a great time for the new employee to clarify any questions or concerns with our administrative team. The new hire checklist is generally completed with the office manager or a senior staff member.

EQUAL EMPLOYMENT OPPORTUNITY:

Our office provides Equal Employment Opportunity to all employees and applicants. Employment decisions are made based on how an individual's skill and qualifications meet the needs and responsibilities of the position for which they have applied or are being considered.

An individual shall not be discriminated against because of race, color, creed, religion, sex age, sexual preference, national origin, citizenship, marital status, disability, veteran status or any other status or characteristic protected under applicable federal, state or local laws. Discrimination and/or harassment based on any to those factors are completely inconsistent with our philosophy of doing business and will not be tolerated at any time.

HARASSMENT:

This office prohibits and discourages any form of harassment, sexual or otherwise. We follow all state and federal employment guidelines regarding such behaviors. Nothing of a sexual nature should be posted, distributed or discussed at our office. Employees should express their feelings if they feel they are ever sexually harassed. Employees are encouraged to contact administration or any of the dentists should any form of sexual harassment occur toward an employee from another employee or patient, or any person in the dental office. Harassment will not be tolerated and is ground for immediate termination. Sexual harassment from a patient directed at a staff member will not be tolerated. The administrative team will review individual cases and if deemed necessary, a patient letter of dismissal will be issued.

PERFORMANCE REVIEWS:

Performance reviews will be performed in the first quarter of every year. Whether or not wage increases are awarded is dependent upon job performance, the office budget and growth within the practice. You may request a performance or wage review at any time. It is the sole discretion of the managing dentist(s) to determine and allocate wage reviews and/or bonus monies as they see fit. There is no guarantee of an annual wage increase of bonus. From time to time, bonus systems will be updated and revised based on the current status and direction of the practice.

Probationary Period/Training Policy:

The first 90 days of employment is a training period for new employees. This is a chance for you to get to know our practice, patients, and professional colleagues. It is also an opportunity for us to get to know you. During the training period, the dentists and practice management will review your work performance and attendance record.

At the successful conclusion of your 90-day training period, you will receive a formal performance evaluation session with our practice manager and one dental partner (dentist). Please note the at-will status of the employees of this practice does not change following a successful completion of the training period. ("At-will" employment status means that either you or the practice is free to end the work relationship without cause or notice at any time during the course of employment.) To help ensure the prompt provision of care to our patients, we request employees who plan to resign to submit letters of resignation with a minimum of two weeks notice.

OFFICE SCHEDULE POLICY:

Office Hours are may fluctuate seasonally but in general are:

Mondays: 7:00-3:00

Tuesday: 8-4:30 (lunch: 12:30-1:30)

Wednesday: 8-4:30 (lunch: 12:30-1:30)

Thursday: 8-4:30 (lunch: 12:30-1:30)

Friday: 8-2pm (No regular scheduled lunch hour)

Our office will close Tuesday-Thursdays between 12:30 and 1:30 for lunch. Be sure telephones are on service before lunch break. Lunchtime is unpaid time off.

*Extra working hours may be available if approved administration, the managing dentist or office manager.

SICK AND EMERGENCY LEAVE POLICY:

A full-time employee is eligible for 3 days of paid sick/emergency leave each year after 90 days of employment. A part-time employee is eligible for 1 day paid sick/emergency leave each year after 90 days of employment. Unused sick leave may not be carried from one calendar year to another. Our office offers a "wellness bonus". At the end of the year, each employee will receive a bonus determined by the administration staff for each unused sick day for which he or she is eligible. Please report your absence as soon as possible for sick/emergency leave.

ATTENDANCE POLICY:

Regular and consistent attendance and promptness are essential for the health and productivity of this dental practice. Please contact the front desk staff if you will be delayed or are unable to come to work due to illness, appointment, or other emergency. The earlier the notification, the easier it is on the office and the rest of the staff. Unreported or excessive tardiness or absences may be subject to disciplinary actions at the discretion of the office manager or managing dentist.

Please arrive 10-15 minutes before scheduled start time to allow enough time to prepare for the day. If you feel you need to arrive earlier to accomplish this, please discuss this with the practice manager. Employees are expected to dress in scrubs or professional business attire, hair neat, teeth brushed, etc. before the first patient arrives. Please also allow 10-30 minutes at the end of the day to finish any daily tasks that allow the office to be prepared for the next day. Be cognizant of patient sensitivities and allergies. Avoid excessive use of perfume or scents.

The office will have regular business hours, however these are subject to change at the Doctors' discretion. We will strive to maintain regular hours and stay on schedule. There may be certain times when this is not possible. Please understand that there will be occasions when you will be required to stay longer than is regular. This is part of the dental health profession and we always need to keep our patients best interest in mind.

Vacation / Personal leave/Holidays:

DEFINITIONS:

*Full time: 4-5 full days. PTO: defined as an 8 hour work day

*Part time: 3 days or less, or half days. PTO: defined as a 4 hour work day

HOLIDAYS: 6 major holidays apply:(Christmas, New Year's, Memorial Day, Fourth of July, Labor Day, and Thanksgiving)

ACCRUED TIME OFF: 1 day per month accrued as working. Days not used may be carried over for one year.

PTO REQUESTS:

Please fill out a PTO request for any PTO you are planning on using. Request slips will be available in a central location gone over during your orientation. PTO requests need to be turned into the practice manager at least one week in advance, (more notice is appreciated!) for approval. Exceptions may be made for emergencies and are subject to approval. Every effort will be made to honor your vacation requests but the practice manager reserves the right to limit the number of staff on vacation at any one time in order to take workload and patient needs into account. In the event of a vacation request conflict, the earliest vacation request submitted will have priority. Calling in sick during a time when a vacation request was denied is frowned upon and may result in disciplinary action, loss of bonus or administrative leave without pay.

DOCTORS TIME OFF:

Doctors will be taking time off for CE, vacation, or family issues. There will be a master calendar located in a central location gone over during your orientation. Great effort will be made to plan far in advance and have dates of Doctor's Time Off listed on this calendar. As you are well aware of, the practice does not function when the dentist(s) are gone for vacation or leave. The office manager will coordinate individual work schedules in the rare instance when all dentists are absent. Specific task may allow staff to work a reduced schedule completing administrative tasks such as ordering supplies, patient recall, approved CE or activities that promote the practice.

*If at all possible please try to arrange any time off for yourself when your Doctor has time off.

*When the Doctor has time off the full time employees have the following options:

1. Use a vacation day

2. Work at other duties as approved by the office manager or Doctor

3. Take the day off without pay

BEREAVEMENT POLICY:

All employees are eligible to take three days off due to a death in the family at a time agreed upon by the dentist. All full-time employees with at least 3 months of employment are eligible to take the three days off with pay at a time agreed upon by the dentist.

Unpaid Time Off:

*In accordance with State law, unpaid time off, up to a minimum of 16 hours annually, is available to all employees who have worked at least one-half time for the previous 12 months, for attendance at school conferences, classroom activities and preschool activities which cannot be scheduled during nonworking hours.

*Time off without pay is available for employees assigned to jury duty upon presentation of the appropriate notice.

*Time off without pay is available for family emergencies, caring for a family member, or maternity leave. These situations will be handled on a case-by-case basis and approved by management.

Voting:

Employees are encouraged to vote and permitted the necessary time off. You will be allowed a reasonable amount of time off to vote.

Overtime:

Full time employees will be paid overtime compensation according to the Fair Labor Standards Act and State laws. When applicable, the usual pay is one and one half of your regular computed wages. You will need prior approval from management in order to work overtime. Sick time and vacation time are not included in overtime hours.

Worker's Compensation:

This dental office carries Worker's Compensation Insurance in accordance to state laws. It is in place to compensate you for any injury, which occurs in the work place. If an injury occurs at work, you are required to fill out an incident report as soon as possible. You may get the report from the office manager. If you experience an injury as a result of your job performance, you are eligible to apply for Worker's Compensation.

DENTAL COVERAGE POLICY:

PREVENTATIVE:

   *No cost to employee or immediate family

SIMPLE RESTORATIVE:

*No cost to employee or immediate family

MAJOR RESTORATIVE:

*Employee and immediate family to cover lab costs

ENDODONTICS:

*Employee and immediate family to cover 35%

*Immediate family is defined as: spouse and dependent children. A case-by-case discount may be given to extended family-to be approved through discussion with the dentist performing the work.

PROFESSIONAL DUES/LICENSING POLICY:

Because our office recognizes the value of professional dental association relationships to your expertise, this practice will pay 100% of dues for one dental-related professional association each year for full-time employees. This practice will also pay for licensing and registration. Please submit your request in writing to the office manager.

CONTINUING EDUCATION POLICY:

Our office holds a strong interest in your professional advancement. Therefore, we will try to attend several continuing education programs as a team. Full-time employees will receive their average daily wage for CE attended as a team. Tuition will be paid for by the practice. Part-time employees will have their tuition paid for the selected CE.

*This office allows up to $200 each year for tuition reimbursement or CE programs for each full-time employee. If you are interested in furthering your professional education in addition to attending the CE programs for the entire team, submit your request in writing to the office manager at least one month in advance. These additional educational opportunities are subject to the approval of the dentist, based on their relevance to your job responsibilities. You will not be paid for time spent in programs.

We will reimburse full-time employees for some CE travel expenses such as meals and hotel charges; the office manager and managing dental partner will approve this on a case-by-case basis. Prior to departure, the office manager must approve travel expenses anticipated for reimbursement. Receipts must be documented, submitted and approved for reimbursement. $30/day is allowed for food reimbursement. Hotel reimbursement is subject to approval and is reimbursed at 50% room rate per full time employee.

SCRUBS:

Our office requires all employees to wear appropriate scrubs or office attire. We will provide scrubs to employees and launder them on-site. Scrub choices

need to be approved by the office
manager. New scrubs will be ordered on
an 'as needed' basis, 3-4 times a year.
Scrubs will be donated or recycled as
they begin to show wear. Our goal is to
maintain a professional appearance at
all times.

EMPLOYEE COMPENSATION:

Our office is required by law to deduct
federal and state taxes as well as Social
Security and Medicare taxes, from every
employee's earnings. By January 31 of
each year, you will be provided a W-2
tax form showing your earnings and
withholdings during the previous year.
Additional deductions may be found on

your paycheck, depending upon your selected benefit package.

MEDICAL BENEFITS:

Details to be determined on an individual basis. Current full time employees are offered coverage at no expense through Blue Cross.

SIMPLE PLAN:

Details to be determined. This plan is available through our financial services consultant and please notify the office manager if you would like further details on this retirement vehicle.

PAYDAY POLICY:

Employees are encouraged to utilize electronic funds transfer for the most efficient payroll process. Paper checks can be issued but the employee understands that these are generated by our accounting firm and can add an additional 2-3 delay in processing and actual receipt of the paycheck for the employee.

EMPLOYEE CONDUCT:

WORK RULES POLICY:

Our office wants to maintain a professional, pleasant, safe, productive, and profitable workplace for you. Most of all, we want you to be happy! These work rules will help maintain this positive work environment. Failure to adhere to these work rules may be cause for discipline, up to and including termination.

*Comply with all safety rules and regulations

*Treat coworkers and patients honestly and ethically. Refrain from unlawful, dishonest, or immoral conduct, including stealing, lying, and falsification of or tampering with records.

*Report to work sober and free from the influence or effects of illicit drugs, alcohol, or controlled substances. You may not possess or use unauthorized controlled substances or alcohol on the job.

*Arrive at work on time and as scheduled, and report back to work on time after scheduled lunch and break times.

*Do not deliberately damage the dental practice's facility, property or reputation.

*Smoking is prohibited in our around our dental facility.

*Please do not conduct personal business on company time. Please limit personal phone calls/texting and emails/computer use.

*Social media may be used if it is for the promotion of the practice or if a specific task related to the use of social media (Facebook, Pinterest, G+, etc.) is assigned by the office manager or dentist.

PERSONAL APPEARANCE POLICY:

CLEANLINESS: Patients judge our adherence to infection control procedures by the personal hygiene of every employee. Daily showers, clean hair, deodorant, and good oral hygiene are recommended fro everyone. Please adhere to moderate use of perfume.

SCRUBS: Scrubs will be worn during patient hours of operation. The practice provides clean scrubs to all clinical staff. Shoes should be well maintained, comfortable and soft soled.

HAIR AND NAILS: In the interest of patient comfort and personal safety, hair should be groomed to stay off the face and out of the way or work. Fingernails should be clean and neatly trimmed.

ACCESSORIES: Visible tattoos and body piercings (besides earrings) are not permitted. Name badges should be worn al all times.

*PERSONAL HABITS: Please do not eat or chew gum in the clinical areas of the office. The entire office is smoke free for employees, patients, and visitors.

CONFIDENTIALITY POLICY / HIPPA:

As dental care professionals, we often have access to personal information about our patients. Information about patients, their treatment or their personal lives must be kept completely confidential.

HIPPA policies are enforced by our management team and also by federal law. If you have questions about confidentiality please ask any of the management staff. When in doubt, always keep patient information confidential.

Be aware of phishing or phone scams as dishonest persons may contact you or the front desk pretending to be an insurance provider and request private information. We have multiple redundant systems in place to prevent identity theft.

*Speak softly or privately with patients so other patients do no overhear.

*Keep the appointment book, case histories, health history forms and other confidential papers, computer screens where patients cannot easily see them.

*Do not discuss the dental treatments or personal information of patients outside the practice.

*Do not reveal information about a patient even to family members without the patient's permission, unless you are speaking to the parents of a patient under age 18.

*Follow all applicable laws covering the release of patient information.

WORKPLACE SAFETY:

All employees will be provided with annual training and review of workplace safety including, but not limited to: OSHA Standards Policy, Blood borne Pathogens Policy, Uniform and PPE maintenance, Hepatitis B Vaccination,

Post-Exposure Evaluation, Standard Precautions, Hazard Communication Standards, Emergency Action Plan Policy and Ergonomics Policy. This training will be done during work hours at no cost to employees.

EMPLOYEE HANDBOOK ACKNOWLEDGEMENT FORM:

My signature on this form acknowledges that I have received a copy of the Employee Handbook. I acknowledge that I have read and understand the contents, and further acknowledge and agree that:

*This handbook is only intended to provide a general overview of our office policies and does not necessarily contain all such policies or practices in force at any particular time.

*This handbook dated

_____, supersedes and replaces any previously written or stated policies or practices covering the same or similar subjects including, but not limited to those contained in manuals, handbooks, correspondence, memoranda or oral discussions.

*Neither this handbook or any other written or unwritten policy or practice this office creates is intended to create an express or implied contract, covenant, promise or representation between this dental office and the employee.

*My employment with this dental office may be terminated at any time, with or without cause or notice by either the Doctor or by me. I understand that I am free to resign at any time.

*I understand that the Doctors reserve the discretion to add, change or rescind any policy or practice ant that any such modification shall not alter the employment at-will relationship. Employees will be notified of any changes to these policies in writing at the time of the change.

_____

_____ Employee

Name (Print)

_____

_____ Employee
Signature

_____

_____ Office staff
reviewing this manual/policies

_____

_____ Date

Dental Practice Resource Group

Job Descriptions

Application

Receptionist/Administr ative Assistant

Reports to: Dr. _____

PRIMARY RESPONSIBILITIES
- Responsible for maintaining appearance and order of dental office
- Patient scheduling
- Patient management

SPECIFIC DUTIES
Reception Management
- - Open and close dental office according to office protocol
- - Check the daily schedule for accuracy and post it in all treatment rooms
- - -Answer and respond to telephone calls with professionalism

- - Review supplies for reception and provide order to business manager
- - Maintain petty cash
- - Ensure that HIPAA Notice of Privacy Practices Notice is on display, if applicable

Patient Management

- - Maintain a professional reception area/office; organize patient education materials, keep the facility neat, etc.
- - Greet and welcome patients and visitors to the practice
- - Check in patients according to office protocol, verifying and updating health information
- - Manage recall and inactive patient system
- - Confirm the next day's appointments by telephone or email or text.- Schedule patients for efficient use of doctor and staff time

- - Check patient back up list to try to fill in cancellation and no-show appointment times
- - Collect payment from patients at time of treatment
- - Make follow-up appointments as needed
- - Assist in the treatment room as needed
- - Records Management
- - Gather and accurately record dental, medical, and insurance information from patients
- - See that records are stored securely and handled in compliance with legal requirements, including the HIPAA privacy and security regulations, if applicable
- - Accurately file patient information
- - Arrange patient charts and radiographs for the next day's appointments
- - Track cases and referrals to and from other doctors

- - Insurance
- - Update insurance information on all patients at all times
- - Submit treatment plans for predetermination of benefits
- - Prepare claim forms for patients with dental insurance
- - Organize supporting materials for claim forms, such as radiographs or written narratives
- - Mail claim forms from office - Assist in the resolution of problems with third-party payers

Billing

- - Prepare billing statements promptly and accurately mail billing statements as directed by the dentist
- - Prepare and mail overdue account letters as directed by the dentist

- - Telephone patients with accounts overdue - Post checks received each day
- - Correspondence
- - Sort, organize, and distribute mail
- - Prepare and send out new patient and referral thank-you letters
- - Prepare and send out continuing care notices on the 15th of each month
- - Prepare and send out correspondence as directed by the doctor
- - Inventory Management
- - Monitor inventory and order dental office supplies as needed
- - Monitor and make sure all dental office equipment is working properly

Office Participation
- - Be an active participant in staff meetings - Perform other tasks as assigned by the dentist

- - Light housekeeping and organization of office to maintain professional appearance throughout and at the end of the day.

PERSONNEL REQUIREMENTS
Education/Experience
- - High school diploma - 2 years' office experience preferred
- - Legible handwriting for notations in schedule

Interpersonal Skills
- - Good interpersonal skills to maintain effective rapport with patients, dentists, other staff members, and community
- - Effective verbal skills to communicate with patients and staff

Lead Assistant: $25-28/hour
Same requirements as above.

Additionally responsible for overseeing the other dental assistants.

Dealing with patient issues and concerns and bringing those concerns to the dentist.

Keeping in perspective the workload for each day and working to coordinate the staff so that work and patients flow smoothly through the practice day.

Tuesday-Thursday: 8:15-4-4:30
Fridays:8-2
BENEFITS
*Healthcare benefit plan: combination plan with a contribution to a health savings account. 90 day trial period
*Simple retirement plan
*Workers comp.
*CE allowance
*Licensing and Registration allowance
*PTO:
  1day/month accrued as working (3 day/year carryover)
   Full time (4 days a week) pd. as an 8 hour day
   Part time (3 days or less/wk.) pd. as a 4 hour day

*Dental Care:
  Preventative: no cost to employee or immediate family
  Simple restorative: no cost to employee
                    Immediate family:
25% of cost
  Major Restorative:
    Employee and Immediate family to cover lab costs
  Endo:
    Employee and Immediate family to cover 35%
Scrub allowance per year.

Dental Assistant

Reports to:

PRIMARY RESPONSIBILITIES
Responsible for assisting the dentist in
the clinical treatment of patients.

SPECIFIC DUTIES

Patient Management
- - Greet patients when they
  sign in and monitor arrival
  time
- - Escort patients to
  treatment room - Seat patients
  and have proper set up for
  procedures
- - Show care and concern,
  and help patients feel
  comfortable
- - Obtain and review health
  histories according to office
  protocol
- - Try not to leave your
  patient unattended in the chair
- - Anticipate and assist
  dentist's needs at all times

- - Perform expanded functions and other tasks as assigned by the dentist
- - Mix dental materials
- - Ensure all patients' questions are answered thoroughly before they leave
- - Chart all patients and record date, service rendered, and any charges
- - Escort patients from the treatment room
- - Ensure proper treatment notes are recorded in patient's chart
- - Perform clinical procedures as practice act allows and as directed by dentist
- - Give patient instruction and demonstrate, when necessary
- - Monitor patient flow
- - Notify Treatment Coordinator if a patient should be called in the evening after a difficult appointment

- - Treatment Room Management and Sterilization
- - Check to ensure that dental units are ready, stocked, and clean at all times
- - Oversee cleanliness of the treatment room according to sterilization procedures
- - Disinfect treatment rooms according to OSHA regulations
- - Sterilize all instruments and hand-pieces according to OSHA regulations
- - Organize trays, instruments, and treatment room drawers at all times
- - Ensure that office sterilization procedures document is on display
- - Send out promptly and monitor all dental laboratory cases
- - Implement a preventative maintenance/cleaning schedule for dental equipment

- - Maintain dental office emergency kits and nitrous and oxygen tanks
- - Follow laboratory procedures according to office protocol
- - Records Management
- - See that records are stored securely and handled in compliance with legal requirements, including the HIPAA privacy and security regulations if applicable
- - Accurately file patient information
- - Arrange patient charts and radiographs for next day's appointments
- - Track cases and referral to and from other doctors
- - Assist in the administration of the recall system
- - Inventory Management
- - Monitor inventory and order dental office supplies as needed

- -   Ensure that treatment rooms are stocked at all times
- -   Office Participation
- -   Help in other areas of the office when necessary (i.e., phones, unpacking supplies, completing insurance forms, moving dismissed patient records, etc.)
- -   Be an active participant in staff meetings - Promote team concept by interacting with others in the office
- -   Light housekeeping and organization of office to maintain professional appearance throughout and at the end of the day.

PERSONNEL REQUIREMENTS

Education/Experience
- -   High school diploma - Graduate of ADA-accredited dental assisting program or

dental assisting experience preferred
- Coursework in dental instruments and procedures
- Compliance with state dental practice requirements (i.e., X-ray requirements, OSHA training)
- Legible handwriting for notations in patient chart; computer skills desired [list programs]
- Commitment to CE for career development

Interpersonal Skills
- • - Good interpersonal skills to maintain effective rapport with patients, dentists, other staff members, and community
- • - Effective verbal skills to communicate with patients and staff

Lead Dental Assistant

Lead Assistant: $25-28/hour
Same requirements as above.
Additionally responsible for overseeing
the other dental assistants.
Dealing with patient issues and concerns
and bringing those concerns to the
dentist.
Keeping in perspective the workload for
each day and working to coordinate the
staff so that work and patients flow
smoothly through the practice day.

BENEFITS

*Healthcare benefit plan: combination
plan with a contribution to a health
savings account. 90-day trial period

*Simple retirement plan

*Workers comp.

*CE allowance

*Licensing and Registration allowance

*PTO:
  1 day/month accrued as working (3 day/year carryover)
  Full time (4 days a week) pd. as an 8 hour day
  Part time (3 days or less/wk.) pd. as a 4 hour day

*Dental Care:
  Preventative: no cost to employee or immediate family
  Simple restorative: no cost to employee
                      Immediate family: 25% of cost
  Major Restorative:
    Employee and immediate family to cover lab costs
  Endo:
    Employee and immediate family to cover 35%

Scrub allowance per year.

Dental Hygienist

PRIMARY RESPONSIBILITIES

- - Comprehensive assessment of patients oral health

- - Review health history in detail

- - Screening procedures including oral cancer screening

- - Take blood pressure if not done by assistant

- - Comprehensive cleaning including SRP

- - Applying sealants and fluoride

- - Patient education

- - Making impressions

- - Promoting the practice and services

Educational Requirements

- - High school diploma and completion of an accredited dental hygiene program.
- - Proof of completion required at time of hire. - Compliance with state dental practice requirements (i.e., X-ray requirements, OSHA training)
- - Legible handwriting for notations in patient chart; computer skills desired [list programs]
- - Commitment to CE for career development

Office Participation

- - Help in other areas of the office when necessary (i.e., phones, unpacking supplies, completing insurance forms, moving dismissed patient records, etc.)
- - Be an active participant in staff meetings - Promote team

concept by interacting with others in the office
- - Light housekeeping and organization of office to maintain professional appearance throughout and at the end of the day.

License

A valid and unrestricted license is required for hire. A copy must be displayed in the office setting at all times. It is the sole responsibility of the hygienist to remain in good standing with state licensure boards.

Interpersonal Skills

- - Good interpersonal skills to maintain effective rapport with patients, dentists, other staff members, and community
- - Effective verbal skills to communicate with patients and staff

BENEFITS

*Healthcare benefit plan: combination plan with a contribution to a health savings account. 90-day trial period

*Simple retirement plan

*Workers comp.

*CE allowance

*Licensing and Registration allowance

*PTO:
  1day/month accrued as working (3 day/year carryover)
  Full time (4 days a week) pd. as an 8 hour day
  Part time (3 days or less/wk.) pd. as a 4 hour day

Dental Care:
  Preventative: no cost to employee or immediate family
  Simple restorative: no cost to employee

Immediate family:
25% of cost
  Major Restorative:
    Employee and immediate family to cover lab costs

  Endo:
    Employee and immediate family to cover 35%

Scrub allowance per year.

Application for Employment

This dental practice does not discriminate against applicants on the basis of race, sex, color, religion, national origin, age, disability, or veteran status. We are an Equal Opportunity Employer.

PERSONAL INFORMATION
Today's Date: _____

Name:_____
_____
_____
_____

Social Security No.:

_____
_____

Telephone:

_____

_____

Address:

_____

_____

_____

_____

Cell:

_____

Email_____

_____

Are you at least 18 years of age?

_____

Are you eligible to work in the U.S.?

_____ Have

you served in the military?

_____

Reserves?_____ Branch?

_____

Have you previously worked at this
practice, or an affiliate?

_____

_____

___
POSITION INFORMATION

Title of
position:_____

_____

Salary Desired:

_____

_____

How did you hear about this position?

_____

_____

_____

Date available for work:

_____

_____

—

Type of work desired (i.e., full time, part
time,
etc.):_____

_____

List special skills, CE coursework, and
experience related to this position:

_____

_____

_____

_____

_____

_____

EDUCATION

High
School:_____
_____
Graduation
Date:_____
_____

Business/Technical:_____
_____Dat
e:_____Degree:
_____
____

College:
_____
_____
_Date:_____Degree:
_____
____

Graduate School:
_____
_____
Date:_____Degree:
_____
____

Additional Skills and Training
_____

_____
_____
_____
_____
_____
_____

WORK HISTORY (Use additional sheets if necessary.)

Company Name:
_____
_____ Address/Phone:
_____
_____ Dates:
_____
_____ Position:
_____
_____ Supervisor:
_____
_____

Pay rate:
_____
_____

Duties:_____
_____

Reason for leaving:
_____
_____

Company Name:

_____

_____ Address/Phone:

_____

_____ Dates:

_____

_____ Position:

_____

_____ Supervisor:

_____

_____

Pay rate:

_____

_____

Duties:_____

_____

Reason for leaving:

_____

_____

Company Name:

_____

_____ Address/Phone:

_____

_____ Dates:

_____

_____ Position:

_____

_____ Supervisor:

_____

_____

Pay rate:

_____

_____

Duties:_____

_____

Reason for leaving:

_____

_____

REFERENCES (Please list three.)

Name:

_____

_____ Years
Acquainted:

_____

_____ Address:

_____

_____ Telephone:

_____

_____

Name:

_____

_____ Years
Acquainted:

_____

_____ Address:

_____

_____ Telephone:

Name: _____

_____ Years
Acquainted: _____

_____ Address: _____

_____ Telephone: _____

_____

PERSONAL

Have you ever been convicted of a felony or criminal offense, including driving under the influence of alcohol or drugs, but excluding minor traffic violations and parking tickets? Applicants are not obligated to disclose sealed or expunged records of conviction or arrest.* A conviction record will not necessarily bar your from employment. Each application will be individually considered on its merits.

If yes, please explain:

_____

_____

_____

_____

_____

_____

_____

_____

_____

_____

_____

_____

_____

_____

_____

_____

EMERGENCY INFORMATION
In case of emergency,
notify:_____

_____

Address:

_____

_____

Telephone:_____

_____

APPLICANT'S STATEMENT (Please read and sign below.) I understand that this employment application and any other Practice documents are not promises of employment. Should I be employed, I understand that my employment will be on a trial period for ninety (90) days from the date of my hiring.* I understand that, if I am employed, I can terminate my employment with or without cause and with or without notice, at any time, and the Practice has a similar right.

I grant permission to the Practice or its duly authorized representatives to contact any persons, companies, schools, or healthcare providers named or referred to in the application (other than my present employer) and I hereby authorize those persons, companies, schools, and healthcare providers to provide my record, reasons for leaving, and all other information they have concerning me to the Practice. I further release all such parties and the Practice from any and all liability claims for damage whatsoever that may result from such contact or information.

The information given by me in this application is true and complete, and I agree that if the information is found to be false or misleading, that I will be disqualified from consideration for employment or subject to immediate dismissal if discovered after I am hired.

Signature of applicant:

_____
_____

Date:

_____
_____

Dental Practice Resource Group

Additional Resources
© 2013 Dental Practice Resource Group

We have included some of our most popular resources below. Please contact us if there is an area of your practice that could use a little assistance. Dental Practice Resource Group has many more resources and this is just a partial list.

We are a multifaceted group. We will listen to your needs and develop a creative solution that works.

Please visit our website for more information:

DentalPracticeResourceGroup.com

If you would like any of our resources in a different format such as PDF or MS Word please let us know. Some of our books and guides are already listed on the website but if you have purchased this comprehensive guide already, please let us know and with a copy of your receipt will be happy to accommodate your request for a different format.

1. OSHA Flow Sheet For Dental Offices

2. Sample Business Plan

3. Employee Review Checklists For All Positions

4. Radiation Safety For The Dental Office

23394467R00051

Made in the USA
Lexington, KY
08 June 2013